The Movements of Gemstone Therapy in the Aura

A Gemstone Therapy Reference Manual

By Isabelle Morton

The Movements of Gemstone Therapy in the Aura
A Gemstone Therapy Reference Manual
By Isabelle Morton

Published by
The Isabelle Morton Gemstone Therapy Institute
P.O. Box 4065
Manchester, CT 06045
U.S.A.
www.GEMFormulas.com

Graphics by Ryan Morton
Edited by Denelle Eknes
Typesetting assistance by AriaRay Brown

IMPORTANT NOTICE

The information in this manual is designed to provide health information for purposes of reference and guidance and to accompany, not replace, the services of a qualified health care practitioner or physician. It is not the intent of the author or publisher to prescribe any substance to cure, mitigate, treat, or prevent any disease. In the event you use this information with or without seeking medical attention, the author and publisher shall not be liable or otherwise responsible for any loss, damage or injury caused or arising out of, directly or indirectly, by the information contained in this manual.

Dedicated to All Who Love Gemstones

Table of Contents

Introducing the Gemstone Therapy
Movements Manual

Welcome to the Gemstone Therapy Institute's *The Movements of Gemstone Therapy in the Aura Reference Manual*, which is designed to accompany my DVD#2 on *The Movements of Gemstone Therapy in the Aura*. Although this manual is available separately, I strongly encourage you to watch the DVD. If a picture speaks a thousand words, a video speaks an encyclopedia. By watching each of these movements on the DVD you can see how they are actually performed. Because there's so much information on the DVD, I felt the manual was essential to have as an easy reference.

The purpose of the DVD and the *Movements Manual* is to help you learn the movements of gemstone therapy and why the body calls for them. When you know what each movement means, you'll have a better understanding of what is going on energetically in the therapy. You can also gain insight into what is happening in the target areas you are working with.

As you become skillful with gemstone therapy, you can use this information to evaluate the energetic picture of a condition, and then, if you are a health-care practitioner, you can make better decisions regarding what other treatments to apply.

I have targeted both the DVD and this manual to energy workers and health care practitioners, and most specifically to gemstone therapy practitioners. In the DVD I used the words "client" and "patient" interchangeably, although technically, gemstone therapy practitioners would have *clients* and professional health practitioners would see *patients*. For consistency, I'll be referring to clients exclusively in this manual.

Although this manual is written for those studying to become gemstone therapy practitioners, those who practice self therapy will also find it a convenient handbook.

Manual Overview

In Chapter 1, I begin with some tips and principles of gemstone therapy that can help you apply gemstones proficiently in the aura. I suggest you read this chapter first.

Chapters 2 through 11 outline each of the movements on the DVD in the order they were demonstrated. Feel free to flip through these randomly as you wish.

In Chapter 12, I discuss the movements that occurred in the real gemstone therapy session that we recorded for Track 12 in the DVD. To get the most from this chapter, watch Track 12 first. Then you may want to watch it again and pause at each section while you read the therapy debriefing that applies.

I end with a glossary so that we're clear about certain terms, which may have slightly different meanings in other schools.

Best wishes on your journey to greater health!

Isabelle Morton
Port Clyde, 8/2010

Chapter 1

Introducing Gemstone Therapy in the Aura

Gemstone therapy involves placing gemstones on the body and applying them in the aura. This manual focuses on the latter. The aura—the energy field that surrounds the body—has a remarkable affinity with gemstone energies. When you present therapeutic-quality gemstones to someone's aura, his or her highest intelligence quickly becomes aware of them. At the same time, the energy field is stimulated by them and begins to interact with them.

If you can hold the gems in such a way that will allow this interaction, you'll find that your client's energy field begins to direct the gemstones to move in certain ways. These movements are archetypical and universal. Everyone's aura moves gemstones in these same basic ways. Moreover, each movement has certain effects and benefits.

These are standard movements that the aura initiates when presented with gemstone energies. They will occur whether you are performing gemstone therapy with mini-gemandalas, custom gemandalas, therapy strands, or necklaces. These movements will also occur if you use other types of energy medicine implements such as energy wands and various types of crystal tools.

The Layers of the Aura
As many of you know, the aura is the energy field that surrounds the physical body. Various schools differ regarding how far from the body the aura extends and how many layers it is comprised of. In gemstone therapy, we recognize 5 primary layers of the aura.

- The supraphysical aura is an approximately 6-inch (15cm) layer of energy that immediately surrounds the body.

- The astral or emotional layer extends another 12 to 18 inches (30cm – 45cm) beyond the supraphysical.

- The causal or memory layer is a little larger than the previous layer and forms a band about 2 feet wide.

- The mental layer of the aura is usually about 3 feet wide.

- The intuitive or subconscious layer of the aura sometimes manifests as a narrow band. But it can also be perceived as a layer that, from a 3-dimensional perspective, seems to extend into infinity.

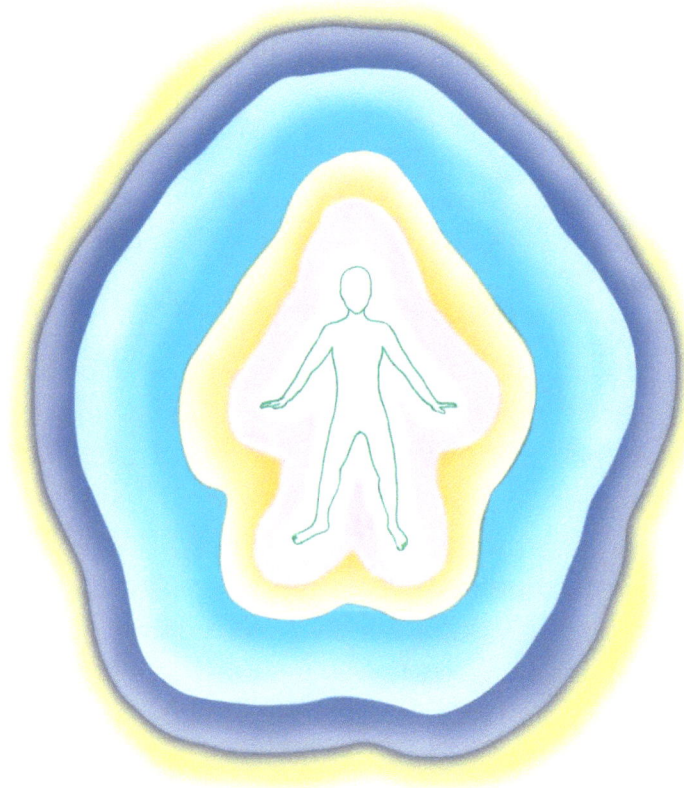

The above graphic of a human aura shows the layers in the following colors: supraphysical-white, emotional-pink, causal-golden yellow/orange, mental-blue, and intuitive-indigo/violet. These colors do not necessarily depict the color that these aura layers appear to be. Instead, they correspond to the colors of the gemstones that vitalize them: supraphysical-White Flash Moonstone, emotional-Morganite, causal-Golden Beryl, mental-Blue Chalcedony, *intuitive-Indigo, (and physical-Emerald).

*As of this publication, the identity of the intuitive body's vitalizing gem has not yet been confirmed.

Tips for Applying a Therapy Rod
A therapy rod is a wooden disk attached
to a round wooden stick. It is used to hold
a mini-gemandala or custom gemandala,
and may even be modified to hold other
types of energy medicine tools.

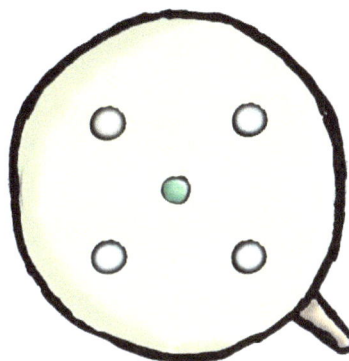

A key to proficient gemstone therapy is
how you hold the therapy rod. You want
to hold the therapy rod in such a way that you
can be most attentive and responsive to the movements your client's energy
field wants to make.

The above graphic shows a mini-gemandala consisting of 4 Mother of Pearl spheres surrounding one Light Green Aventurine sphere. The gems are attached to the disk with modeling beeswax.

Here are some tips for proficient use of a therapy rod:

- Always hold the therapy rod so that it is pointing directly to the center of the anatomy you are working on. I call this "pointing to the bone." I demonstrated this in DVD#1 on *Mini-Gemandalas for Self-Therapy*. The graphics shown on the chapter title pages illustrate a proper orientation of the therapy rod in relation to the body.

- Hold the therapy rod lightly, with just enough pressure in your fingers to keep it from falling. Don't squeeze the rod or tighten your hand muscles unnecessarily.

- Your fingers, hand, arm, and shoulder should be relaxed while you apply the rod. If you start to tire, work with your other hand.

- You can hold the rod with either your right or left hand, or both.

Tips for Enhancing Your Sensitivity to the Aura's Energies
When you hold a therapy rod in someone's aura, the aura will initiate energy
flows that the gemstones on the rod will want to ride upon. Here are some
ways to enhance your sensitivity to these flows so that the gems can follow
them with ease:

- Hold an attitude of curiosity and watchfulness during a therapy session. Observe what happens to the gems in the client's aura. Witness what is happening, as though you are completely uninvolved. This can help you to avoid controlling the movements or initiating them on your own.

- Put your attention on listening and you'll know instinctively what the body is asking for. Although you may not hear anything, the practice of listening puts you in the state of mind that allows your body to respond intuitively to the aura's energy flows.

- Look at the part of your client's body where the movements are centered, but also use your peripheral vision so that you are always attentive to the person's entire being. By giving attention to your peripheral vision, you will more likely be able to perceive the energies in your client's body and how the gemstones are interacting with them.

- Try not to think about the movements that are occurring. Remember, *you* don't perform or direct the movements. You're only the vehicle for supporting the gemstones so that they can ride the body's energy flows.

- Do your best to be as sensitive as possible to any movements you may feel. Trust yourself and your intuition. Once you get how it feels when the aura moves gemstones, it's a skill you'll be unable to forget.

- Be as attentive as possible to the gemstone therapy you are providing. If personal thoughts arise, set them aside without criticizing yourself. Keep your attitude positive as you simply continue to give your full focus to the session.

Respecting Your Client's Aura
The principles of gemstone therapy support a relationship of respect and trust between you as a practitioner and your gemstone therapy client. These principles include:

- If you begin a therapy session, continue to apply the gemstones until your client's energy field is finished with them and signals that it is time to end the therapy. (In Chapter 11, I'll describe what these signals are, and also how to gracefully end a therapy cycle if time is running short.)

- Respect your client's energy field by giving it the movements it wants and allows. Trust yourself to be the best vehicle you can be to perform these movements.

- Do not intentionally force movements. By doing so:

  - You can violate any relationship of trust that you've developed with your client's energy field. This trust is essential. With it, your client's energy field will open and initiate movements. Without it, your client's energy field can begin to resist you and put up protective mechanisms.

  - You can disrupt your client's energy flows. Only the client's higher intelligence knows what movements are best, and the perfect priority of their application. If you intentionally force a movement, you can encourage energy to move in a wrong direction, open flows the body isn't ready to receive, and disperse energy from areas that need it. This can cause further weakness or gather energy to areas that already have an excess, thus contributing to any imbalances that may already be there. Furthermore, you can encourage the release and transfer of information the body isn't ready to handle or look at.

- If your heart is sincere, and you're not intending to give the body movements it doesn't want, then don't worry that you're doing something wrong. Enjoy the healing session, as it will uplift both you and your client in many ways.

> Just because we cannot see the body's energies doesn't mean they do not exist. With the advent of many types of energy medicine modalities today, more practitioners are aware of how to sense and palpate these energies. Gemstone therapy allows you to work with these energies directly. By observing the pathways the gems take, we can actually see and interact with the aura's energy currents.

Practicing the Movements

Because it is not appropriate to perform movements that the aura has not asked for, practice them using a blank therapy rod and perform them over an inanimate object, such as a pillow.

In the making of DVD#2, *Movements of Gemstone Therapy in the Aura,* I could not demonstrate each movement on a real person because at the time I wanted to show you a particular movement, my client's aura may not have wanted it. So, I demonstrated on a large doll named Sally. My family gave me mixed feedback about whether or not I should have used Sally. But demonstrating the movements over a pillow instead seemed much less "real." I hope you will accept Sally in the spirit of good humor in which I presented her.

Notes:

Chapter 2

The Pull In, Ease In, and Cushion

Before a gemstone therapy can begin, your client's aura has to accept the gemstone energies. It does this by drawing the gems toward the body with either a pull in or an ease in movement.

The Pull In™

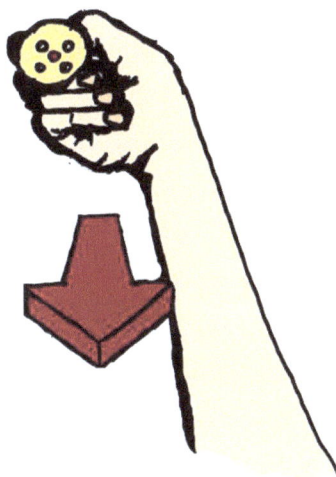

What Is a Pull In?
A pull in occurs when the body's energy field wants the energies of the therapeutic gemstones that are presented to it. In this case it will directly draw the gemstones to itself in a relatively straight line. This is a pull in.

How the Pull In Occurs:
When you hold therapeutic gemstones in the aura and are ready to start a gemstone therapy session, your client's higher intelligence will evaluate the gemstone energies. If it clearly and definitely wants them, it will initiate a

magnetic-like draw that pulls the gems toward your client's body. In general, the more receptive the body's energy is and the more it needs these gemstone energies, the stronger the pull in is likely to be.

- If the energy field has yet to learn the effects of the gemstones being presented, the pull in may be relatively weak. Or, an ease in movement will draw the gems instead.

- When you feel a pull in, allow the client's energy field to draw the gemstones toward the client's body. A pause may occur before another movement begins—usually circling.

- If you feel a particularly strong pull in, rein it in somewhat so that you don't bump the body with the gemstones. Stop an inch or two (2.5cm to 5cm) above the surface of the body. If the pull in persists, gently touch the body with the gems. Then perform movements appropriate when a therapy rod is touching the body, like pressing or tapping (see Chapter 8). Or, the rod may lift up a little and being spinning or unlocking (Chapter 6), or proceed to do the touching movement (Chapter 9). Or, it may lift up even further and begin circling (Chapter 3).

The Pull In Movement:

- Can occur over any area of the body.

- May stop and start again as the gems move toward the body, sometimes pausing a moment at each level of the aura.

- Can also occur during a session—and not just at the beginning. If you're working in a higher layer of the aura, the body's energy may use a pull in to move the gemstones closer to the body.

The Purpose of the Pull In:

- To let you know that the body's energy field is ready to receive the gemstones you are ready to apply.

- To give you a relative sense of how receptive the body's energy field is. A strong pull in means it is very receptive. A weaker pull in means it is less ready or doesn't yet fully understand the benefits the gemstone energies can offer.

- Sometimes a pull in will identify a target area that you may or may not be aware needs healing attention. Subsequent movements will center around that area to uplift it.

Notes:

Notes:

The Ease In™

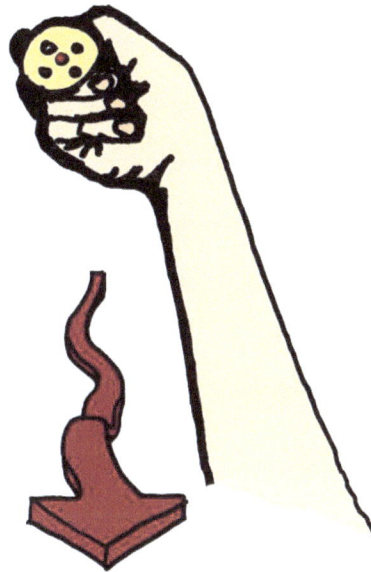

What Is an Ease In?

The ease in may occur instead of a pull in at the beginning of a gemstone therapy session. It may occur if your client's energy isn't sure about the energies of the gemstones being presented to it or how to receive them, or if it isn't sure exactly where therapy should start.

How the Ease In Occurs:

The gemstones will trace a meandering path toward the body and around it until they find an entry window. At this point, the energy field will accept the gemstones and begin to move them in the archetypical movements of gemstone therapy.

While the ease in is happening, remain open minded and allow the gems to follow whatever path the body's energy is leading them on. Any doubt you may feel is probably not your own. You may just be picking up that feeling from your client's energy field, as it tries to decide how to receive the gemstones being offered.

The Ease In Movement:

- May continue for several seconds or as long as a minute or two.

- Can guide the gemstones toward the body along a path that is not straight or direct.

- Can move the gemstones in a meandering path that may run up and down the body until the body's energy finally begins to move the gems in an archetypical way.

The Purpose of the Ease In:

- To help the body get to know the energies of the gemstones you are applying.

- To give the body time to decide how to accept the gemstone energies and where to direct them.

The pull in and ease in are the two types of movements that begin a gemstone therapy session. Pull ins are directed to target areas. An ease in can occur whether or not a specific area is targeted for therapy.

Notes:

The Cushion™

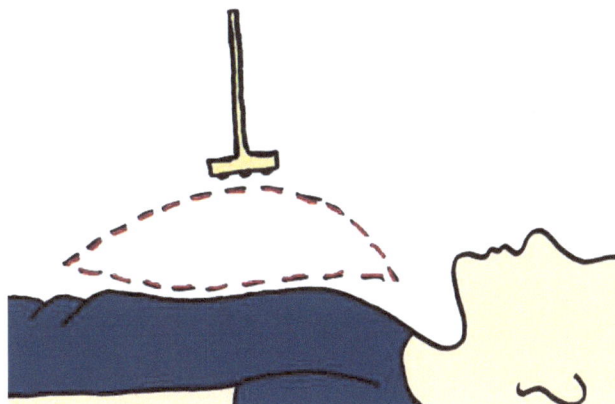

What Is a Cushion?

A cushion is a pillow of energy the body produces to protect itself against gemstone energies that it does not feel ready for, or that it knows would be incompatible at this time.

How a Cushion Occurs:

When you are presenting gemstones to the aura, a pull in or ease in may lead to a cushion of energy that prevents the gemstones from moving any closer to the body. This means that you should apply the gems in the aura above the cushion. If you bounce the gems against a cushion repeatedly, it will probably grow stronger. If you ignore the cushion, and try to apply the gems closer to the body than the body wants them to be, you may feel a growing sense of discomfort, usually in your heart or stomach.

The Cushion:

- Usually occurs at the start of a therapy to let you know at what layer of the aura the body wants the gems to be applied.

- Can occur during a therapy when you have not responded to a push away or let go.

- Should be considered a welcomed indicator. Its presence assures us that the body knows what it needs and what it does not.

If you have selected gemstones that your client's energy field has asked for (such as when selecting a mini-gemandala or making a custom gemandala), and the cushion occurs over a target area, the body may be asking for a different entry window.

If you present gems simply because they are the next in a series (such as in a mini-gemandala pack) or because you'd like to try a therapy with a certain pre-designed gemandala, then it may be that the entire body isn't compatible with those gems at this time. To find out if this is the case, try approaching the body from different points and see if you get a cushion at these areas, too.

The Purpose of the Cushion:
The body's energy will form a cushion to guide you to perform the gemstone therapy in a certain layer of the aura, or to protect itself against gemstone energies it doesn't want or need. In most cases cushions are unmistakable, so beginners shouldn't worry if they aren't sensing one.

To learn what a pull in, ease in, and cushion feel like,
practice them on yourself.

Find a comfortable position sitting or standing. Take a deep breath and center yourself. Randomly select among the therapeutic-quality gemstone necklaces or GEMFormulas remedies in your pharmacy. Hold your selection in your hand, at arm's length in front of your chest.

Invite the gemstone energies into your energy field. Gently prompt them to begin moving toward the center of your chest, just above your heart. As the gems approach your body, be sensitive to their response. Does your body accept them and draw them in? Or do you feel a slight resistance or cushioning sensation?

A relatively strong movement of the gems toward your body is a pull in. It feels as though your body really wants the energies of the gemstones. If the gems slowly meander to your body, that's called an ease in. Now honor your energy field: If you're holding a necklace, put it around your neck; if you selected a GEMFormulas remedy, take a dose.

If you sense some cushioning, it means that your body is not open to these gems at this time. Note what the cushion feels like.

Chapter 3

Circling, Spiraling In, Spiraling Out

Circling™

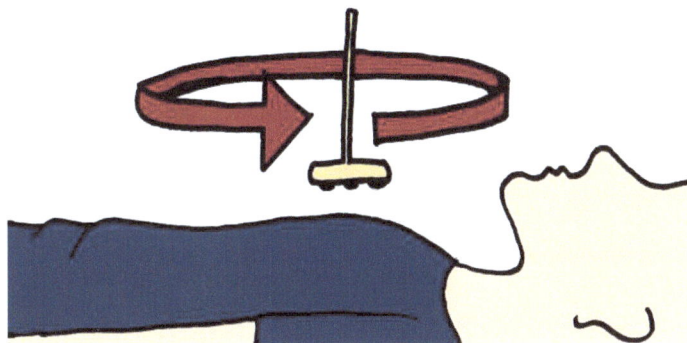

What Is Circling?

Circling is a basic movement that usually begins every gemstone therapy session. It may also be performed as a transition from one movement to another.

How Circling Occurs:

When you perform a circling movement, the therapy rod moves in a round shape that is parallel to the surface of the body. Circles typically repeat. You could do an entire gemstone therapy just using the circling movement.

Circling is typically the first movement the body will ask for. In addition, the body often returns to circling after you perform other movements.

Sometimes the circling movement is shaped like an oval, such as when you are encompassing both knees at the same time, or working along the length of a limb, or when addressing adjacent body parts such as the wrist and elbow. (If you targeted the wrist or elbow by itself, the shape would more likely be a true circle.) When chakras call for circling, be sure the shape is as round as possible.

The Circling Movement:

- Can be performed over any area of the body.

- Can consist of circles of any size. They can be large enough to encompass the entire body or as small as an inch (2.5cm) in diameter.

- Can move clockwise or counterclockwise, as the body's energy prefers.

The Purposes of Circling:

- Foremost, circling helps to gather, process, and integrate information about the area over which the movement is being performed.

- Secondly, circling helps the body's higher intelligence decide what movements to guide the gemstones to do next.

Other purposes of circling:

- To teach the body about the nature and benefits of the gemstones being applied.

- To establish an energetic connection between the gems and the body.

- To provide an opportunity for the client's highest intelligence to develop trust and build a relationship with the practitioner.

- To help the client's body gather information about the organs, tissues, cells, molecules, atoms, plus the emotions, karma, thoughts, concepts, excess energies, deficiencies, resources, and so on that exist within the circle being made.

- To communicate the information gathered within the circle to the body's higher intelligence.

- To help the body evaluate what has happened during previous movements (and decide what movements to do next).

- To help the body process and integrate all the work that has been done so far. Circling can provide a rest period between other movements.

Spiraling In™

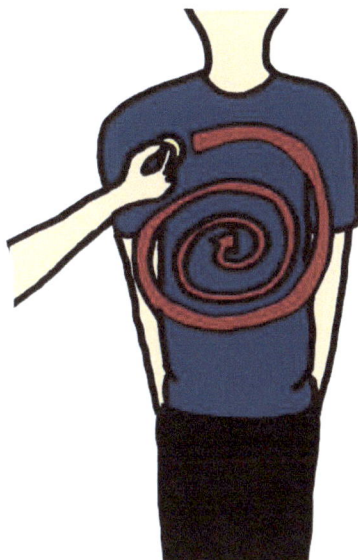

What Is Spiraling In?

The spiraling in movement is an outcome of circling. After the body's energy field has gathered information during the circling movement, it may then want the gemstones to help it guide this information toward a target point. This target point exists in the center of the spiral in.

How Spiraling In Occurs:

When you perform a spiraling in movement, the gemstones follow a circle that gets smaller and smaller until they reach a point or a very small circle. When you reach that point:

- A spiraling out movement may occur, followed by another spiraling in movement, and so forth.

- The gems may go directly back to the outermost perimeter of the spiral and then immediately repeat the spiraling in motion.

- A movement typical to individual points may occur, such as spinning, unlocking, or plunging.

The Spiraling In Movement:

- Can occur over chakras, organs, and target areas.

- Can go clockwise or counterclockwise.

- Can repeat many times or occur just once.

- May or may not be associated with the spiraling out movement.

The Purpose of Spiraling In:

- During the spiraling in movement, information that has been gathered from the tissues and cells in the outer perimeter of the spiral is transported to and communicated with the tissues and cells in the center of the spiral.

- This movement also collects and concentrates gemstone energy at the target point.

Notes:

Spiraling Out™

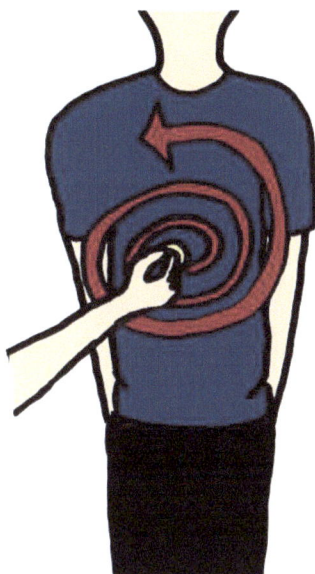

What Is Spiraling Out?

The spiraling out movement is often an outcome of movements performed over a target point. These movements include spinning, unlocking, tapping, holding, and plunging. After these movements have released information or excess energy, the body may need this information broadcast over a larger area or dissipated. The spiraling out movement accomplishes this.

How Spiraling Out Occurs:

When you perform a spiraling out movement, the gemstones move from a central point outward, in circles that gradually expand in size. When you reach the perimeter, a few movements can then happen.

- A spiraling in movement may occur, followed by another spiraling out, and so forth.

- The gems may go directly back to the target point and then immediately repeat the spiraling out motion.

- Or a different movement may occur, such as circling or vortexing.

The Spiraling Out Movement:

- Is usually associated with a target point.

- Can go clockwise or counterclockwise.

- Can repeat many times or occur just once.

- May or may not be associated with the spiraling in movement.

The Purpose of Spiraling Out:
The spiraling out movement is the opposite of the spiraling in movement.

- During a spiraling out, information in the central target organ is communicated with the tissues in the outer-lying areas of the spiral.

- Excess energy in the central target organ is spread out and dissipated.

When Spiraling In and Spiraling Out Repeat:
When spiraling in and spiraling out alternate, a great deal of therapy occurs as information and energy are brought to the spiral's center and unwanted energy is released and distributed for eventual dissipation. The more often these two movements repeat, the deeper into the target organ the gemstone energies can get. The deeper they get, the more information or excess energy the target organ can release, and the more healing energy it can receive.

Notes:

Chapter 4

Vortexing In, Vortexing Out, and Columning

The movements described in the previous chapter take place on a flat plane and are considered two-dimensional movements. The vortexing in, vortexing out, and columning movements are each three-dimensional movements.

The vortexing movement technically consists of two separate movements called vortexing in and vortexing out. Although these two movements are often performed repeatedly one after the other, each has a different energetic purpose, and so I'll explain them separately.

The vortexing movements are usually performed over chakra centers. Sometimes areas that are experiencing pain or disharmony create a vortex in the presence of gemstone energies in order to aid their healing process. So, if the gemstones start moving in a vortex over an area of the body that is not a chakra center, you may want to pursue other types of evaluation at that area.

When doing the vortexing movements, the gems trace the shape of a cone. When columning, they trace the shape of a coil or spring.

Vortexing In™

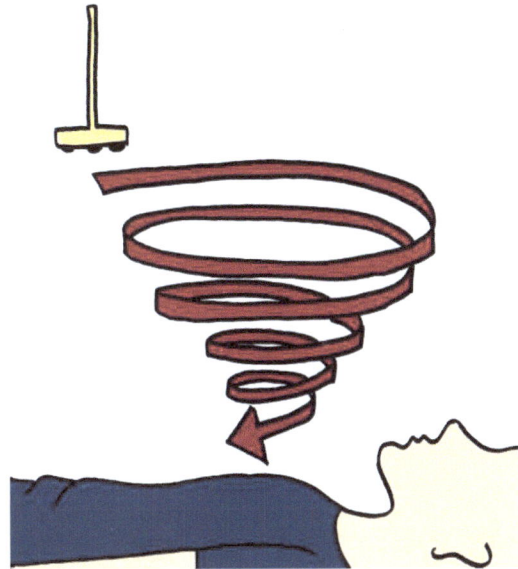

What Is Vortexing In?

Vortexing in is a three-dimensional movement that takes place in one or more layers of the aura. The movement traces the natural conical flow typical of chakra centers and local energy vortices.

How Vortexing In Occurs:

Vortexing in usually begins with a circle some distance from the body. When the circles start to become smaller and also move closer to the body, then you know that the gemstones are following a natural vortex flow and you are making a vortexing in movement.

The vortexing in movement is almost always followed by the vortexing out movement. However, it may instead be followed by another movement.

The Vortexing In Movement:

- May be performed over chakras, organs, and target areas.

- Can go clockwise or counterclockwise, as the body's energy prefers.

- Gives you a sense of how well energies are moving into and nourishing the body, by how definitely and quickly the gemstones follow the vortexing in movement.

The Purpose of Vortexing In:

- To strengthen the energetic structure of a chakra vortex so that it can function more effectively.

- To repair weaknesses in a chakra vortex.

- To nourish the target area with healing energies from the aura.

- To convey to the rest of the body the directional nature of the chakra's vortex. Upon evaluation, the body may decide to test the alternative direction, in which case if the gems have been moving clockwise, the body's energy may have them move counterclockwise and vice versa. If this is the case, you may experience a half vortex (see Chapter 5) until the body's energy decides upon a direction.

- Vortexing in can also let you know where an actual energy vortex is located on the body. A healthy body will construct a temporary vortex to aid the healing of a target area.

Notes:

Vortexing Out™

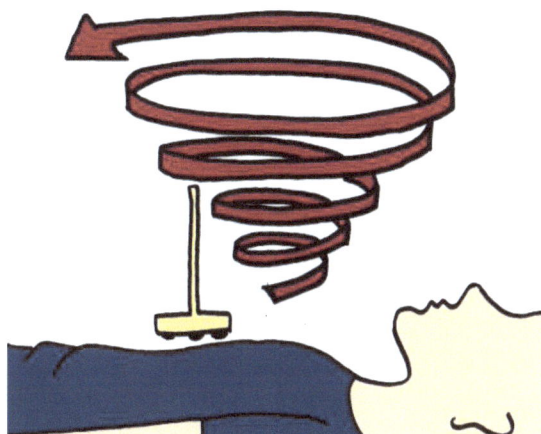

What Is Vortexing Out?
Vortexing out is also a three-dimensional movement that takes place in one or more layers of the aura and typically over chakra centers.

How Vortexing Out Occurs:
This movement begins at a point or at a very small circle performed near the body. You'll know you're doing a vortexing-out movement when the very small circles begin to increase in diameter at the same time as they move away from the body.

The Vortexing Out Movement:

- May be performed over chakras, organs, and target areas.

- Can go clockwise or counterclockwise, as the body's energy prefers.

- Shows you weaknesses in the chakra vortex by inconsistencies or anomalies in the gems' movement as it traces the vortex.

- Gives you a sense of chakra health by showing you how far into the aura a chakra vortex is extending.

The Purpose of Vortexing Out:

- To encourage a vortex to grow in size, strength, and reach.

- To correct the shape of weakened or deformed vortexes.

- To share information contained in the target area, such as the state of its health, with the target area's counterparts in the aura and subtle bodies.

Note: A common indication of chakra weakness is a short chakra vortex. Ideally, a healthy chakra vortex should extend through all layers of the aura. If the gems reveal a shortened vortex, you can invite your client's higher intelligence to take notice. Doing so can have an immediate impact on the vortexing out movement. Each time you repeat the vortexing in/vortexing out sequence, the vortexing out movement can grow longer as it traces a chakra vortex that is being restored. (Practitioner 1 students learn other ways to support the lengthening and strengthening of chakra vortexes.)

Notes:

Columning™

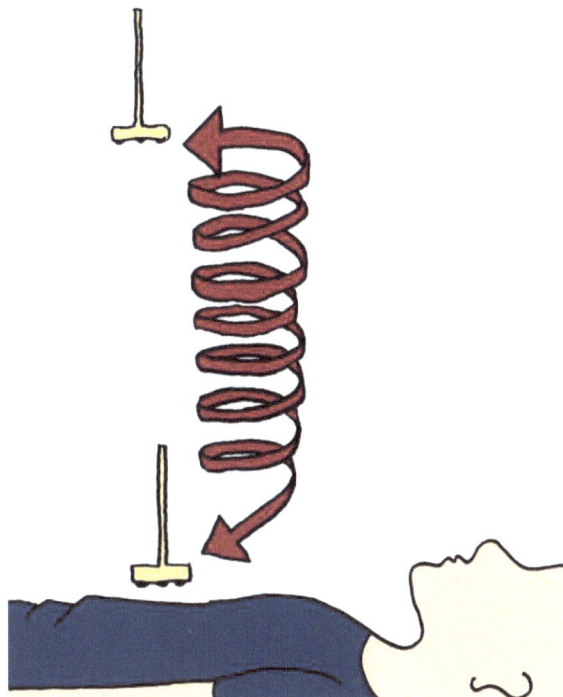

What is Columning?

Columning is a 3-dimensional movement that spans more than one layer of the aura. When you do this movement, the gems trace the shape of a coil or spring.

How Columning Occurs:

The columning movement begins as a circling movement. If the circling starts near the body, it will suddenly telescope upward to form the coil shape. If the circling begins away from the body, the column will extend downward.

The Columning Movement:

- Can go clockwise or counterclockwise.

- Can range in diameter from about 2 inches (5cm) to about 10 inches (25cm). Small-diameter columning may occur if you are working over a small part of the body such as an eye or an injury in a small area. Columning of a larger diameter may occur over a visceral organ, such as the stomach, or another relatively large part of the body, such as a shoulder or hip.

- Can vary in length. It can span a mere foot (30cm) into the aura, or it can reach as far into the aura as your arm can reach.

The Purpose of Columning:

Columning is called for when the body's intelligence wants the gemstone energies to help make a connection between a physical organ and its energetic counterparts in the aura. Once this connection is made, the columning movement then provides a way for information and energies to pass back and forth between these counterparts to align and harmonize them, and to reconcile excesses and deficiencies.

Note: The columning movement can occur vertically or horizontally in relation to the body. The graphic on the previous page shows a columning movement in a vertical orientation, which is "pointing to the bone." Horizontal columning is oriented parallel to the spine. It usually takes place along the body's midline and supports the client's personal vortex.

Notes:

Chapter 5

Half Circling, Half Spiraling, and Half Vortexing

The half circling, half spiraling, and half vortexing movements are transition movements. They usually occur when the energy flow of a circle, spiral, or vortex is about to change its direction.

Directional changes are significant. They signal that a decision is in the process of being made or they indicate a shift is about to happen in some aspect of a client's life. This could include her outlook, attitude, feelings, or beliefs. It can also result in a desire to make different, healthier choices, which can lead to change in her "direction" in life, her interactions with others, and how she regards herself.

Half Circling™

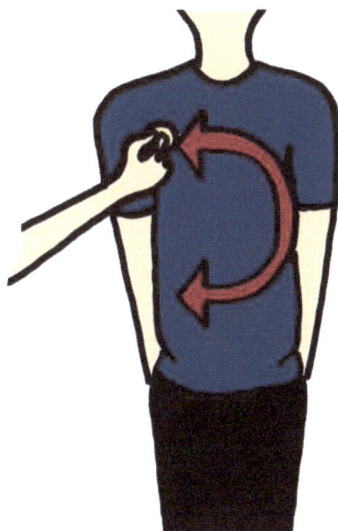

What Is Half Circling?
Half circling is a transition movement that signals a change in the direction of a circling movement. It involves the retracement of an arc of the circle's perimeter.

How Half Circling Occurs:

Half circling occurs when you are performing a circling movement and the gemstones stop, move briefly in the opposite direction, stop, and then move briefly in the original direction, and on and on until circling resumes in either direction.

The half-circling movement looks as though it is retracing a portion of the circle's perimeter.

The Half Circling Movement:

- May continue for two or more retracements of the arc.

- May last as long as a minute or two, but usually lasts only about 10 to 20 seconds.

- May occur at various speeds, which may also change as the body is evaluating in which direction to continue the circling movement.

- Can retrace any portion of the circle. This portion may be one-half of the circle as pictured in the graphic on the previous page, or a smaller arc, or one that spans as much as three-quarters of the circle.

During half circling, the gems may pause briefly each time they are about to retrace the arc in the opposite direction.

The Purpose of Half Circling:

- To signal that the body is considering a change the direction of the circling movement.

- To help the body decide in which direction the circling movement should proceed.

Half Spiraling™

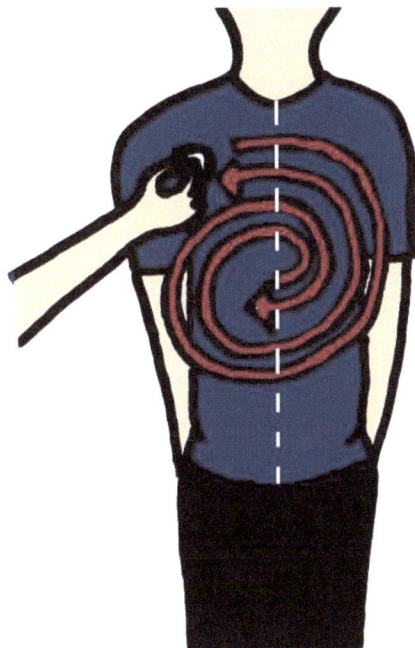

What Is Half Spiraling?

Half spiraling is a movement that signals that a change in the direction of a spiraling movement may occur. As the gems retrace the shape of a half spiral, the body's intelligence decides whether or not to make this change.

How Half Spiraling Occurs:

You'll know you're doing a half spiral when the gems start making a spiral in or spiral out movement, but stop and then retrace a small portion of the spiral shape, stop, and then retrace that same portion once again. The gems may repeatedly retrace the arc until the spiral either continues in the same direction or changes directions.

The Half Spiraling Movement:

- Usually occurs after you've been doing a spiraling movement.

- May lead to another spiraling in or spiraling out, which would go in the opposite direction or the same direction.

- Can continue for two or more retracements.

- Can occur at various speeds.

- Can retrace any size portion of the spiral, but usually no more than one-and-a-half full turns.

During half spiraling, the gems may pause briefly each time they are about to retrace a portion of the spiral.

The Purpose of Half Spiraling

- To give the body's intelligence a chance to evaluate the effects of the previous spiral direction, and decide if it wants to continue in that direction or change it.

- To alternately spread and collect information in order to prompt an energy shift or improvement in energy flows to the area.

Notes:

Half Vortexing™

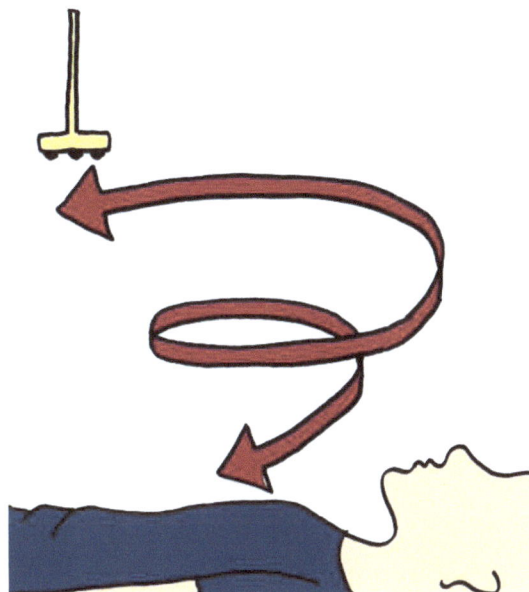

What Is Half Vortexing?
Half vortexing is a movement that signals a change in the direction of a chakra vortex.

How Half Vortexing Occurs:
Half vortexing occurs when you are doing a vortex in or vortex out movement and the gemstones stop, retrace a portion of the vortex, stop, and retrace the same portion once again. This will continue until the vortexing movement continues in its original clockwise or counterclockwise direction or changes its direction.

Because the switch of a chakra vortex's direction can mean significant changes in a person's life, pay careful attention when you follow a half vortexing movement.

The Half Vortexing Movement:

- Occurs over major or minor chakra centers or wherever energy vortexes are found on the body.

- Can continue for two or more retracements.

- Can occur at various speeds.

- Usually retraces no more than one-and-a-half full turns, but can retrace any size portion of the vortex.

- Can retrace different sections of the vortex. For example at first you may retrace the vortex in the emotional layer of the aura, and then immediately afterward retrace portions of the vortex in the causal or mental layer of the aura.

During half vortexing, the gems may pause briefly each time they are about to retrace a portion of the vortex shape.

The Purpose of Half Vortexing:

- To help your client's body decide which vortex direction is most supportive and harmonious.

- To help the body make the directional shift in a chakra vortex.

Notes:

Chapter 6

Spinning, Unlocking

Here are two movements that occur over a single target point.

Spinning™

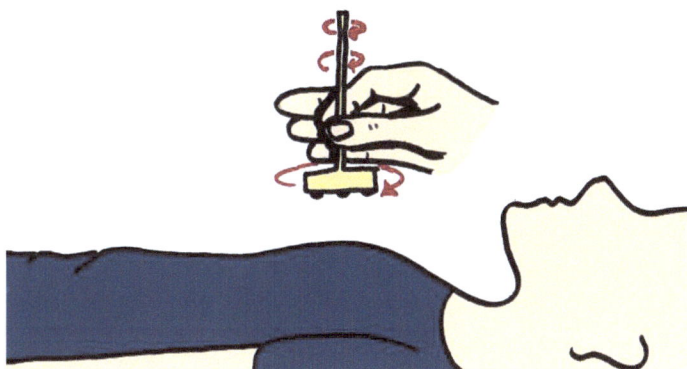

What Is Spinning?
Spinning occurs with the therapy rod pointing to a target point. The spinning movement is usually one of a series of movements that take place over that target point.

How Spinning Occurs:
When you spin a therapy rod, you move it in one direction only. Always maintain control of the spinning movement. If the spinning momentum takes over, you may find yourself spinning the therapy rod so fast that you lose connection with your client's energy field. If this occurs, the spinning is no longer effective. Therapeutic benefits only occur when you maintain a connection to your client's energy field.

The Spinning Movement:

- Can occur clockwise or counterclockwise.

- Change directions one or more times before the client's energy field initiates a different movement.

- Take place at any distance from the body.

- Can occur at the same time as other movements, such as circling or plunging.

- Can happen slowly or quickly.

- Usually requires 2 hands to perform.

The Purpose of Spinning:

- Spinning has a vacuum-like action that draws out built-up energy from within a target point.

- Spinning dissipates built-up energy that is ready to be released.

Notes:

Unlocking™

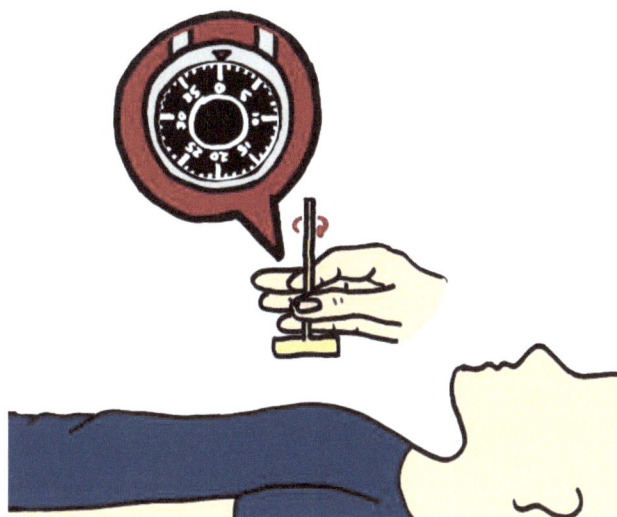

What Is Unlocking?

Unlocking is a means to release unwanted energies trapped within a target point.

How Unlocking Occurs:

The Unlocking movement occurs over a single target point. The therapy rod remains pointing to one spot on the body, as in spinning. But instead of making many turns in one direction only, the therapy rod moves back and forth to varying degrees. When you perform the unlocking movement, the motion feels similar to unlocking a combination safe.

The Unlocking Movement:

- Can occur within the aura at any distance from the body, or as close to the body's surface as possible.

- Can happen slowly or quickly.

- Can occur at the same time as other movements, such as circling or plunging.

- Can consist of relatively large turns back and forth, or tiny micro-turns that can seem barely perceptible.

To get the most benefit from the unlocking movement, pay close attention to the connection between the gems on the therapy rod and the body's energy. Be as sensitive as you possibly can to the unlocking. The more precise the unlocking motion, the more effective it will be.

The Purpose of Unlocking:
Unlocking offers several benefits. It helps to:

- Release blockages of stuck and stagnant energy to open energy flows.

- Enhance energy flows already in motion but sluggish.

- Release the energies of emotions, memories, or thoughts that may be stuck in the target point and negatively affecting its health.

- Release information about the target point so that the body's intelligence can take another step in the healing process, including what next movement to ask for.

- Release accumulated and excess unwanted energy from the target point.

Notes:

Chapter 7

Jiggling, Holding, and Plunging

Here are three more movements that may occur in the aura over a single target point. Let's start with a movement that I call "jiggling."

Jiggling™

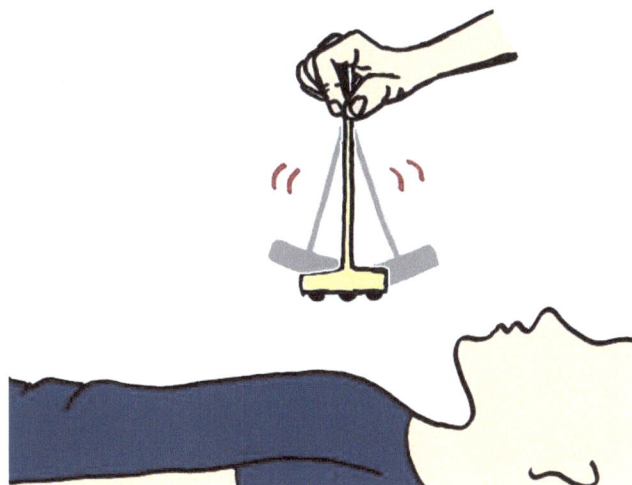

What Is Jiggling?
Jiggling is a movement that signals that the gemstones, while moving in the aura, have located an area of disturbance. Unlike a blockage, which is stuck energy, disturbances in the aura relate to energies that are conflicting or interfering in some way.

How Jiggling Occurs:
Jiggling occurs when a therapy rod starts to shake, or jiggle, while you are applying it. If it occurs during a circling movement, it is usually limited to one portion of the circle. It will feel as though the pathway that the gems take over this portion is bumpy, while the rest of the circle is smooth.

Be aware of the jiggling, but just keep performing the circle (or other movement), and invariably the disturbing energies that are causing the jiggling will be resolved.

If they are not resolved by the movement of the gems alone, try squirting some GEMFormulas' Energy Clearing Spray in the area where the jiggling is taking place.

The Jiggling Movement:

- Usually occurs while other movements are being performed, such as circling or spiraling.

- May occur over a single target point.

- Can appear suddenly while you are working on an area.

The Purpose of Jiggling:
The purpose of jiggling is to signal the body's intelligence that an area of disturbance has been located. By continuing to give the area gemstone therapy, the jiggling usually subsides as the gemstone energies reconcile the jagged frequencies and smooth them out.

Notes:

Holding™

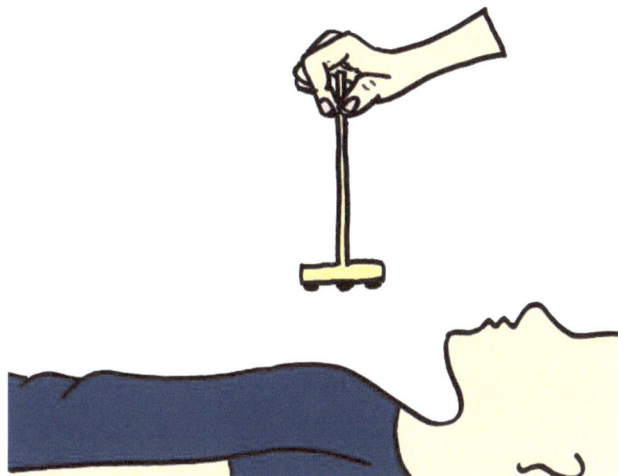

What Is Holding?

Holding is actually no movement at all. It occurs when the gemstone energies have facilitated a significant amount of change in the energy field, and the body needs some time to incorporate these shifts. Holding often leads to a "still point," which is a deeper, more reflective state. During a still point, information is evaluated, examined, processed, and integrated, and therapeutic changes are made.

When holding begins, the body decides if it wants to go more deeply into a still point, or just continue processing the information at a relatively superficial level.

How Holding Occurs:

During a holding, the therapy rod stops over a target point. The body's aura gives no indication that it wants to move the gems, push them away, or let them go.

The key to a successful holding is to maintain the energetic connection between the body and the gemstones. One way to do this is to hold your free hand with palm facing the therapy rod at a comfortable distance. The energy will build between your hand and the therapy rod.

Holding can be challenging for beginners because it seems as though nothing is happening. If you are unsure, you can prompt another movement every 5 to 10 seconds by gently urging an unlocking, plunging, or circling motion.

If you gently try to urge another movement and you still feel as though an elastic band is keeping the gemstones in place, then the holding is still effective.

The Holding Movement Can:

- Occur when the therapy rod suddenly stops.

- Result from a gradual slow-down of a movement that ends in a halt.

- Last for a few seconds or for as long as a minute. Once again, if a holding lasts longer than this and you aren't sure if you've lost the connection or not, test it by prompting another movement.

- Occur when actually touching the body, although it usually occurs in the aura.

- Look exactly like a still point, but a still point is deeper, and draws you in with a sense of purpose and intensity.

The Purpose of Holding:

- To help the target point over which the holding occurs to integrate the shifts that have recently occurred during the gemstone therapy session.

- To prepare the body to receive more gemstone therapy.

- To provide a gateway for a still point, during which healing changes are made. During a still point, the body accepts, processes, and integrates the work in a deeper, more profound way, often encompassing many levels of being.

Plunging™

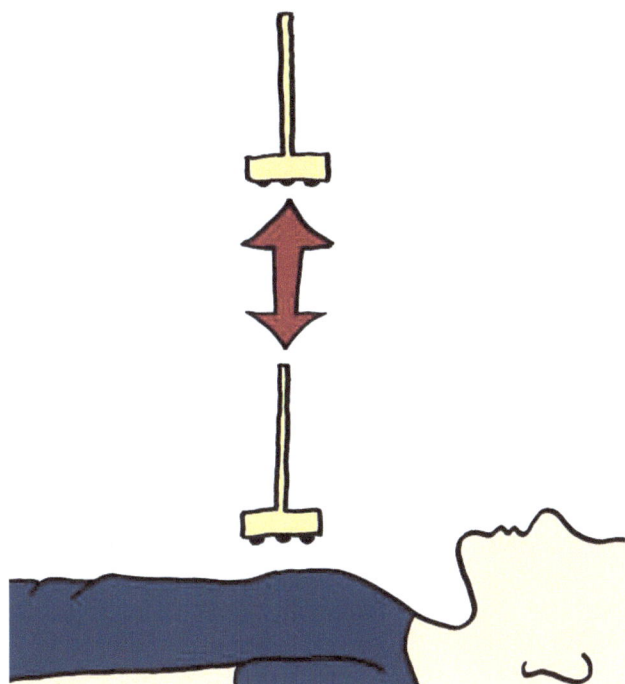

What Is Plunging?

Plunging occurs over a single target point and resembles a pumping motion.

How Plunging Occurs:

Keep the therapy rod pointing to the target point and move the rod toward and away from the body in a straight line.

The Plunging Movement:

- Can occur at any distance from the body. It can be very close or relatively far away in the aura.

- Can retrace a relatively short, straight line of only a few inches (8cm), or a relatively long one of about 12 to 18 inches (30cm to 45cm). Most plunging movements are less than a foot (30cm) long.

The Purpose of Plunging:

- The plunging movement can occur when the target point needs to be energetically massaged before it can let go deeply rooted energies that it has been holding onto.

- It can also serve to prime the pump, so to speak, by filling the target area with gemstone energy. This can give it the support it needs to let go of unwanted energy.

Notes:

Chapter 8

Pressing, Tapping

During a therapy session, it's possible that the therapy rod will touch the body and not want to leave. This could be a holding movement, as previously discussed. However, if it lasts more than a few seconds, you should consciously call to mind the pressing and tapping movements to see if the body's energy field wants them. Simply think about the movement and then see if your client's energy responds by guiding the gems to perform either one.

Pressing™

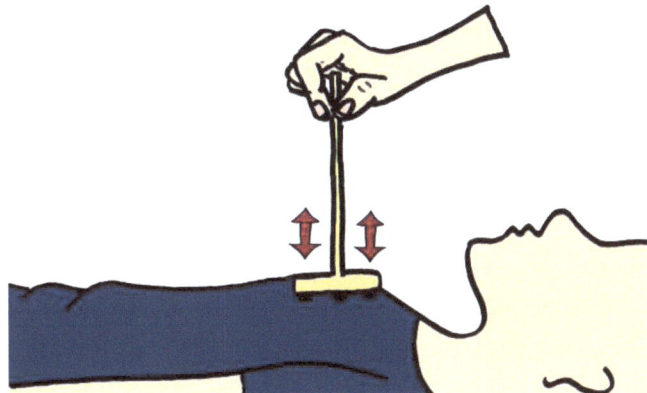

What Is Pressing?
Pressing occurs while the therapy rod is touching a target point. When you do this movement, you simply press the therapy rod gently into the skin.

Pressing is the body's way of getting the gems to make contact with a layer of tissue at or beneath the skin. This is called establishing rapport.

How Pressing Occurs:

While holding the therapy rod against the skin, slowly and gently press the rod into the skin until you sense rapport. When you find it, it will feel as though a deeper connection or sense of relationship has been established between the gemstones, the client's body, and yourself as the practitioner.

Once you have found this rapport, the gems might continue with a holding movement. Or they may do a micro-plunging. In this case, you gently release and reapply pressure on the therapy rod.

Pay careful attention when the body calls for pressing because the movement can be subtle.

The Pressing Movement:

- May be barely perceptible to an observer, but the client can usually feel it.

- Can be intense if you hold the gems at the desired level of rapport. Energy will build until you get a push away or the gems do a different movement.

- May be followed by holding, micro-plunging, or micro-unlocking movements.

The Purpose of Pressing:

- To bring the gemstone energies into a deeper physical level of the body. You might say this movement allows them to penetrate the skin to work inside the body itself, and to contact the energy flows that exist just underneath the skin.

- Another purpose of pressing is to allow the gemstone energies to find a greater level of rapport with the target point so that further therapy in the aura will be more effective, especially for the organs and tissues associated with that target point.

Tapping™

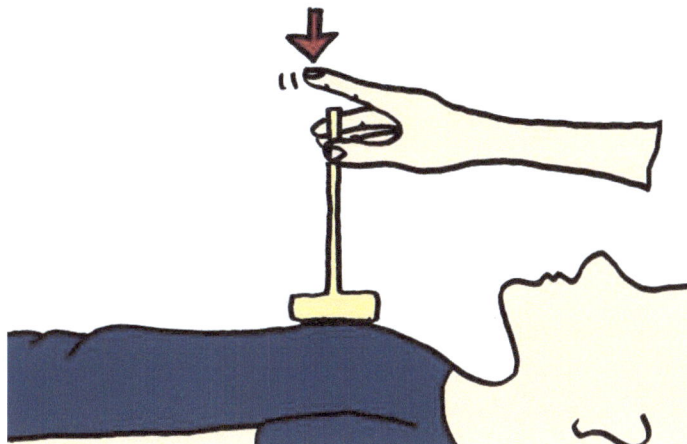

What Is Tapping?
Like a pebble dropped into a pond, tapping initiates a wave-like motion that can radiate information about the target point throughout the body.

How Tapping Occurs:
With the therapy rod touching the body, gently tap the end of the rod with your finger two or three times. If this does not initiate a push away or let go, or initiate a different movement, repeat the tapping.

The Tapping Movement:
Tapping should be performed gently. Sometimes the more gently you can tap, the more effective the movement will be.

The Purpose of Tapping:

- To inform the body that the target point needs healing attention.

- To wake up the target point, so that it becomes more self-aware and more cognizant of what it needs to improve its health.

- To stimulate the target point, so that it can reveal its needs, or to recognize that it has been holding onto unwanted energies, which it might then release.

Notes:

Chapter 9

The Figure 8, Multiple 8, and Touching

In this chapter I'd like to describe three common movements that involve more than one target area of the body. These are the figure 8, the multiple 8, and touching. Each of these movements unites the target areas in some way, usually by enhancing communication or distributing information or energies between them.

The Figure 8™

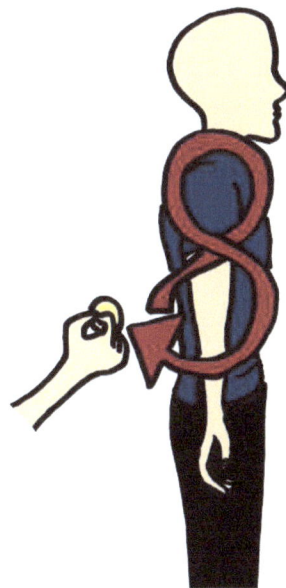

What Is the Figure 8?
The Figure 8 is a movement that encompasses two target areas.

How the Figure 8 Occurs:
The movement usually begins with circling. The therapy rod suddenly breaks away from the circle to start another, adjacent circle going in the opposite direction. Instead of closing this second circle, however, the rod retraces the first circle, and so on.

The Figure 8 Movement:

- Can link any two organs or target areas of the body. These two areas may or may not be adjacent to each other, but they are usually within the same body section.

- Links organs or areas that are energetically associated with each other in some way.

- Can repeat once or twice, or many times. Usually the more times it repeats, the more the two target organs need to share information and/or energy with each other.

If the figure 8 repeats many times, you may want to further investigate the state of health of the two target organs.

The Purpose of the Figure 8 Movement:

- To let you know that two organs are somehow involved with each other energetically. Perhaps they're sharing or borrowing energy from each other, or perhaps there's a breakdown in communication or function between them.

- To correct energetic imbalances between the two organs. Inappropriately shared energies can be returned, miscommunications can be corrected, and ties of limiting energy can be released.

The Multiple 8™

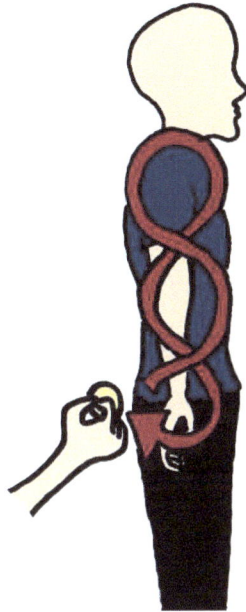

What is the Multiple 8?

A multiple 8 is an extension of a figure 8, but 3 or more target areas are involved.

How the Multiple 8 Occurs:

The Multiple 8 usually begins as a wavy line that extends along the body. When the gems return to retrace the wavy line, they instead move opposite each previously-made curve to create the multiple 8 pattern.

The Multiple 8 Movement:

- Can involve 3 or more target areas that will be adjacent to each other, such as the wrist, elbow, and shoulder.

- When performed over the spine, it can consist of many small ovals linked together, as the gemstones crisscross over individual vertebra or groups of vertebra.

- Can be repeated a few times or many times.

The Purpose of the Multiple 8:
Like the figure 8, this movement lets you know that the target areas encompassed by the multiple 8 are somehow involved with each other energetically. By performing the multiple 8 movement, corrections can be made in any energy imbalances, miscommunications, misalignments, or improper ties between these target areas.

At the same time, the multiple 8 unites the target areas in some way, usually by enhancing communication and shared energy flows, or distributing or redistributing energy between them.

Notes:

Touching™

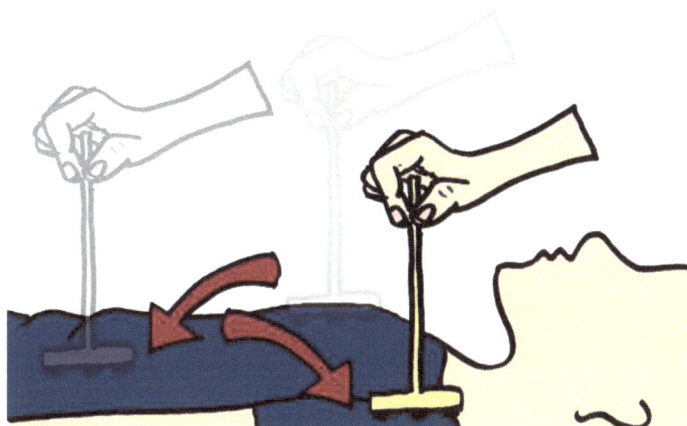

What Is Touching?

The touching movement connects target areas by simply touching the body at a series of target points.

How Touching Occurs:

This movement can take you by surprise. You can be circling, spiraling, or doing any other movement, and suddenly the therapy rod is drawn to touch down on the body. Touching usually lasts only a few seconds.

The difference between holding and touching is that holding usually lasts much longer and involves only one target point. With touching, the gemstones move from point to point.

Note the target areas where touching occurs because they are invariably linked together. If touching repeats over these areas, you may want to examine their health more closely using other diagnostic methods. For example if you notice that touching occurs over endocrine glands, you may want to look into the health of your client's endocrine system and support it in some additional way.

The Touching Movement:

- May involve two or more points.

- May move from point to point along a path that seems random.

- May alternate between two or more points repeatedly.

Furthermore, the therapy rod can move directly from one touch point to another, or meander from one point to the next, or perform a circling movement between touch points.

Touching may also involve points in the aura that correspond to physical points. In this case, the touching movement proceeds exactly as it otherwise would, although the gems stop in the aura. Usually (but not necessarily) this takes place within 6 to 8 inches (15cm – 20cm) of the body.

The Purpose of the Touching Movement:

- To alert the body's higher intelligence that an energetic connection exists between the target points involved in the touching movement.

- The organs and tissues associated with the touched points can become aware of their relationship with each other.

- To transfer information or energies from one touched point to the next.

Notes:

Chapter 10

Meridian Running, Striping, and Vertical Circling

In this chapter I'd like to describe three movements that work with the body's acupuncture meridians and energy flows. We'll start with meridian running.

Meridian Running™

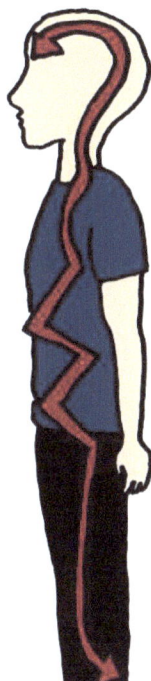

What Is Meridian Running?

Meridian running is a movement that involves tracing an acupuncture meridian with the therapy rod. If you are familiar with the acupuncture meridians, your meridian running can be quite accurate. However, you don't need to know anything at all about the meridians for the body's energy to move the gemstones in a linear way up and/or down the body.

How Meridian Running Occurs:

Sometimes gemstones will move in an uninterrupted path from the beginning of a meridian to its end. More often, however, when an area of sluggish energy is located, the gems will move back and forth, retracing a small portion of the meridian line until it is cleared. The gems will then proceed farther along the meridian and do more meridian running, or become involved in an entirely different movement.

Let's say you knew nothing about the meridians in your client's arm. But her body's energy is aware that there is a blockage in one of them that needs clearing. Without even knowing about the meridians, you may be drawn to do meridian running up and down her arm.

However, if you did know that the lung meridian started inside the front of the shoulder and ran down the arm to the thumb, then you could more accurately move the gems along this exact energetic pathway.

The Meridian Running Movement:

- Can run the entire meridian once from beginning to end.

- Can initiate repeated retracing over one portion of a particular meridian or several portions of that same meridian.

The Purpose of Meridian Running:

- To clear blockages or sluggish energy in a meridian line.

- To revitalize the energy flows in that meridian line.

Notes:

Striping™

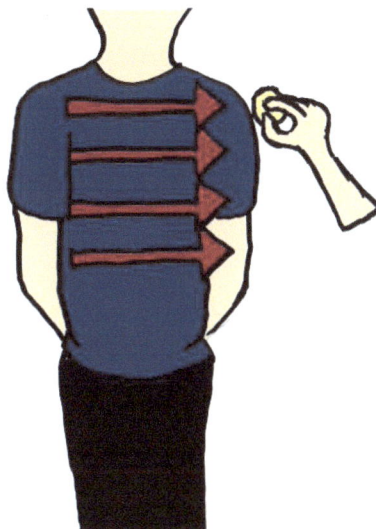

What Is Striping?

While meridian running clears blockages or sluggish energy along one line, striping clears blockages or sluggish energy over an entire area.

How Striping Occurs:

Striping often begins as meridian running, but shifts into a two dimensional movement as the portion of the meridian run is replicated to the left or right, about one-half inch (about 1cm) or more from the original line. The result is a striping movement that involves tracing and retracing parallel lines over the target area.

The Striping Movement:

- May appear to be moving energy back and forth, but actually there is a distinct direction involved. To encourage this direction, trace the striping line close to the body. Then lift the therapy rod a little ways away from the body when the rod returns to start a new line.

- May occur just once, in which case the therapy rod traces each line only one time. Or the therapy rod may retrace the stripes many times.

- May trace lines that are perpendicular to the spine, as shown in the graphic, or ones that are parallel to the spine.

- May or may not be associated with actual acupuncture meridian lines.

The Purpose of the Striping Movement:
The purpose of this movement is to clear sluggish energy over a wide area. Although it may appear that the gems are working only on the surface of the body, their energies are penetrating it to whatever depth they are needed.

Notes:

Vertical Circling™

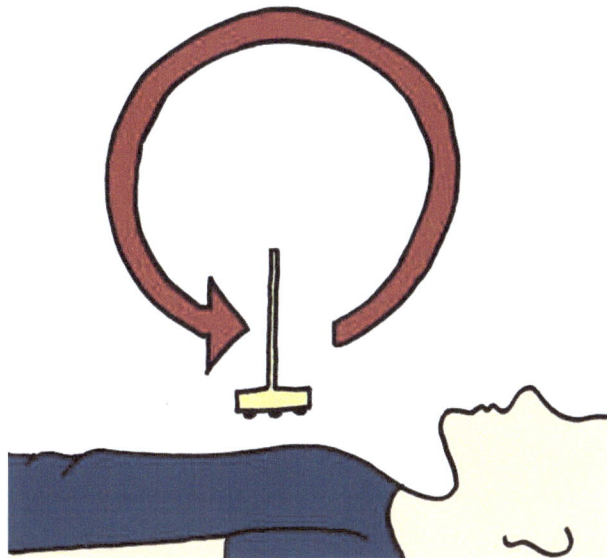

What Is Vertical Circling?
Vertical circling also moves energy along meridian lines, but does so not just physically. A vertical circle also engages the supraphysical counterparts of the meridian.

How Vertical Circling Occurs:
Instead of the quintessential circling described in chapter 3, which occurs on a plane parallel to the surface of the body, a vertical circle moves upright in relationship to the body.

The Vertical Circling Movement:

- Tends to follow meridian lines or energy flows.

- Usually encompasses the supraphysical aura, which means the circle is about 6 to 8 inches (15cm to 20cm) in diameter, although it could be larger or smaller.

- Can move energy up or down the body as needed. The above graphic shows a vertical circle moving energy up the body.

- Usually occurs relatively close to the body and parallel to the spine if applied to the torso, or parallel to a limb if applied to the arms or legs.

- Can sometimes occur perpendicular to the body's midline. In this case, it may be strengthening your client's personal vortex.

- Tends to be stronger than meridian running because of the momentum produced by the circling movement.

The Purpose of Vertical Circling:
To strengthen energy flows. In comparison, meridian running tends to open blockages and relieve sluggishness in meridians, although it can also vitalize them. Vertical circling often follows meridian running. After the meridians are clear, their flows often need to be fortified both physically and supraphysically.

Notes:

Chapter 11

The Push Away and Let Go

When a therapy cycle is complete, your client's energies will let you know by releasing the gemstones from his or her aura. This can occur in two basic ways, one is called the push away and the other, the let go. These are called completion movements because they signal that a therapy cycle is finished. After you get a push away or a let go, you can end the therapy session completely. Or, if time allows, initiate another therapy cycle by adding another gemstone to the custom gemandala, or work with a different gemstone necklace or mini-gemandala.

The Push Away™

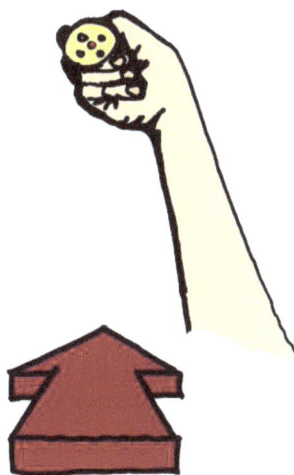

What Is the Push Away?
The push away is the more dramatic of the two completion movements. Your client's energy field will literally push the gemstones that you are holding, out of his or her aura.

How the Push Away Occurs:
When a push away occurs, whatever other movement you have been doing will stop, and your therapy rod will move directly out of your client's aura. The push away is a definite movement that's hard to miss.

The Push Away:

- Can occur after any amount of time has passed during a session. A person's energy field may gain all it can from certain gems within a minute or an hour. In some cases, you can anticipate a push away when the movements slow down. But not always.

- If you are nearing the end of the time allowed for a therapy session and your client's energy field shows no signs that she is finished with a particular gemstone, then it's possible to remind her energy field of the agreed-upon therapy duration. Do this by talking to your client with your thoughts or aloud. Simply let her know how many minutes she has left in the session. Invariably this will initiate a graceful push away or let go.

The Purpose of the Push Away:
The push away signals it is time to end a therapy cycle and to remove the gemstones from your client's aura.

Notes:

The Let Go™

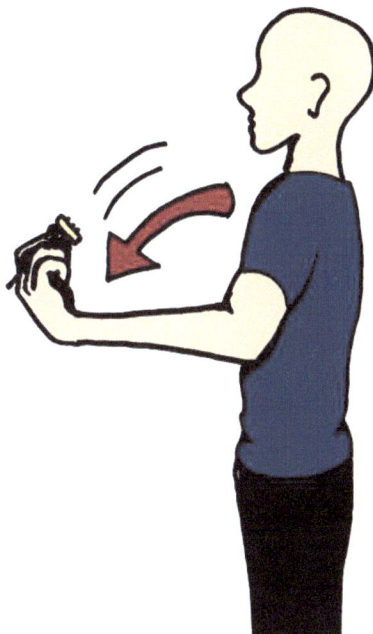

What Is a Let Go?
The let go is another way that your client's energy field can signal the end of a therapy cycle or session.

How the Let Go Occurs:
After performing any number of other movements, you may suddenly no longer feel any urge to move the gems at all. The energetic connection between the gemstones and your client's energy field dissolves and disappears, but no definite push away occurs. This is called a let go.

Don't be tempted to think that the lack of further movements is your fault, or that you have done something to lose the connection with your client's energy field. This is not the case. If you feel you've lost the connection, accept it as a true let go. Remove the gems from the aura. If time permits, add another gemstone to the custom gemandala or offer a different gemstone therapy tool.

The Let Go:
Like the push away, a let go can occur at any time during a session. Within a minute or an hour your client's body may gain all it needs from the particular gemstones you are applying.

The Purpose of the Let Go:

The let go signals that your client's body has probably had enough of the energies provided by the gemstones you are presently applying, but it may not be absolutely sure it is completely finished with them.

The let go is less definite than a push away. When you get a push away, the body's energy field is quite certain that it doesn't want the gemstones that you've been applying any more. But with a let go, the body's energy field is less certain. Therefore, if you get a let go, keep in mind that your client's energy field may again want these gemstones later on in the session. Therefore, if you are applying a gemandala, do not disassemble it when you get a let go, as you may need it again soon.

Notes:

Chapter 12

The Movements in Therapy

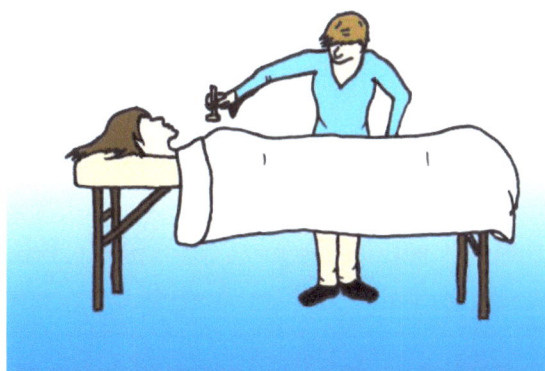

In this chapter, I'll share an in-depth debriefing of the real-life gemstone therapy session that you saw in Track 12 of DVD#2 *The Movements of Gemstone Therapy in the Aura*. This explanation should give you a better understanding of how the movements of gemstone therapy come together. You may wish to review Track 12 while reading this section, and then put the player on pause periodically to read about what you've just seen.

The Therapy Begins
Prior to filming, I performed the initial steps of the basic gemstone therapy protocol. The Foundation Five necklaces were placed underneath the sheet that was covering my client's body. Since the filming, I've learned it's best to put the necklaces above the sheet. They work just as effectively, and much of the unwanted energies they draw off the body are dissipated into the aura instead of being absorbed. Then they'll need a less intensive cleansing afterward.

In this session, we used all 4 gems in the Mini-Gemandala Pack for Physical Healing. In these mini-gemandalas, 4 Mother of Pearl surround a central gemstone. These central gems are: Light Green Aventurine, Dark Green Aventurine, Chrysoprase, and Green Tourmaline. I had set up each of these mini-gemandalas beforehand so I wouldn't have to interrupt the therapy session to change the central gemstone.

About Intention

For this recording, I specifically asked my client *not* to discuss any conditions with me beforehand. We wanted to demonstrate how the gemstones can locate target areas on their own, which they did. Of course, to get the best and the most from a gemstone therapy session, it helps if your client states an intention, or in other words, a goal for the session.

- If an intention involves a specific target organ or area (e.g. the stomach), you can begin a gemstone therapy by holding your mini-gemandala nearby that area, and waiting for a pull in or ease in.

- If there is no intention stated prior to your session (or if the intention defines no single or identifiable target area), then start as I did in Track 12. I held the therapy rod in the aura above the shoulder, slowly moved it toward the body, and allowed the body's energy to choose an entry window.

Building a Relationship Between Body and Gems

As you watch this gemstone therapy session, notice how slowly the gemstones come in. Likely this was because my client was receiving her first gemstone therapy session and her energy field was tentative. Her higher intelligence was taking time to get to know the gemstone energies. By respecting this slow ease in, we allowed a relationship to build between the gemstones and my client's body. We also took a step toward building trust between her higher intelligence and myself as the practitioner.

At first, I did not feel a significant connection between the gems and my client's energy field. Nevertheless, the gems kept moving. They moved according to how my client's energy wanted them. When the therapy rod started moving down my client's body and to her legs, the connection and the relationship started to build. The connection continued to be strong as the therapy rod moved up the body using the touching movement.

Note how this touching movement did not make physical contact with the body. That's okay. It was building bridges of communication between each corresponding part of the body that the movement targeted.

By the time the therapy rod began working on my client's head, I felt that her energy field finally understood what the gemstones could do. You can see how the movements became faster and more definite.

Work at My Client's Head Begins
Some circling over the head followed by circling over the heart indicated a transfer of energy from the head to the heart, or communication between them. I sensed my client's body was trying to redistribute the weight that was on her mind, and to help her let go burdensome thoughts.

Then we had a columning movement over her head that extended into her aura. This is another way to distribute information, and reduce the weight of energy on the physical tissue. Because the columning occurred over the head, I assumed it was also helping to relieve weighty thoughts.

Looking back, we had two movements that signaled too much energy in my client's head. This could mean she was over-thinking a problem, or that she had a disharmonious process going on within her skull. We would find out if the gems would give us any other clues.

Next, we had some brief holding over the top of her head. At this time, her higher intelligence was trying to figure out what to do next. It was as though it was saying: "The accumulation of excess energy in the head has been identified. It's been somewhat smoothed out, transferred somewhat to the heart, and spread through the aura through the columning movement. But how should we guide the gems now?"

Unlocking
The subsequent unlocking motion happened through the levels of her aura, and this told me that her physical and subtle bodies were well connected. All were aware of what was going on with her health, but wanted deeper information to be uncovered. The unlocking motion revealed more of this information.

As a result of this information coming forward, I was able perceive the place inside her head where the gems were connecting, and I mentioned this on the recording. The unlocking also revealed that the source of the surplus energy may have been excessive thinking to some extent, but more importantly, there was actual disharmony going on in the brain itself.

Soon after the unlocking, we got our first pull away. It was as though the body was saying: "Okay, we have identified a significant target area with Light Green Aventurine. Now let's use Dark Green Aventurine to take this a step further."

Transitioning From One Mini-Gemandala to Another
When a mini-gemandala or custom gemandala leaves the body or aura, remember the location, and make sure to bring in the next one at this same location. This way your application is seamless.

In the case of this client, the Light Green Aventurine/Mother of Pearl exited out the crown chakra. So this is where we brought in the Dark Green Aventurine/ Mother of Pearl mini-gemandala.

Focus on the Brain
The Dark Green Aventurine/Mother of Pearl mini-gemandala came in easily, but I always wait and watch for a relationship to develop between the gems and the target area. In this case, it seemed to occur right away.

The brain tissue asked for various types of movements. Because some of these movements occurred in the causal aura, it hinted that there may have been a karmic or past-experience connection to her present condition.

How Are You Doing?
At some point during a treatment session you may have the urge to ask your client how she is doing. When I word the question this way, I usually get a simple answer: "I'm fine."

If you are focusing treatment at a particular area, you might say, "Can you tell me what's going on right now in your [name the area]." You're more likely to get a more specific answer this way.

In this particular session, I asked how my patient was doing because there was a lot of treatment focusing on her head. The head can pick up gemstone energies very well, and sometimes people can become lightheaded. Asking them how they're doing is a simple way to get them back in touch with their body and acknowledge what's going on. It actually helps them to process any work that you are doing inside the head.

My client acknowledged that she was having trouble with her pituitary gland, and that she was forgetting things. Later on, she explained that this had become a significant disability.

Alert Your Client to the Gemstone Touching Movement
Also note that I alerted my client before I touched her head, so as not to surprise her. Your clients may have their eyes closed and may not know where you are working in their aura. For this reason, it's nice to let them know where the therapy rod wants to touch down.

My client mentioned that the touching was making her head tingle more, but I checked for balance and everything seemed okay. To check for balance, I simply asked in my thoughts if the gems being used were okay for her, and although I could sense everything was okay, I muscle-tested with my fingers to allow my mind to verify my knowing.

Later on, I thought we had a push away, but the gems just wanted to be further away from her body. Then it suddenly felt as though the "elastic band" feeling between the gems and her head simply disappeared. This is a classic let go.

Starting the Next Mini-Gemandala at the Exit Window
The Dark Green Aventurine/Mother of Pearl mini-gemandala exited near the crown chakra, so that is where we brought in the next mini-gemandala. The Chrysoprase/Mother of Pearl mini-gemandala gave us a classic pull in, directly over her pituitary gland at her forehead.

I was drawn to perform some circling movements. I mentioned these circles were working at the back of her head and the first two vertebrae at the top of her neck. How did I know that? Because when you apply the gemstones, it feels like there is an elastic band or some sort of energetic connection between the gems and the target area. All I had to do was follow this "elastic band" to the target area and identify the anatomy that the gems were connected to.

The more you know about anatomy, the more accurately you can distinguish what parts of the body the gemstones are working on. It's possible to become very specific—even to identify certain tissue layers in some cases.

Using Energy Clearing Spray
Then we connected with some very stuck, frozen energy in her neck. I applied the Energy Clearing Spray. This was an excellent demonstration of how quickly and efficiently the Energy Clearing Spray can dissolve unwanted energy and allow treatment to continue. Otherwise, you'd have to work through the stuckness, which can take a significantly longer amount of time. Note how much smoother the movements became.

Take note of the circling down the left side of her body. It was probably helping the rest of her body to integrate the work that we had done at her head. The circles were systematically collecting energy and moving it down her leg, and then back up again.

Working with Chrysoprase

I usually keep the therapy table lower than I might if I were a massage therapist, simply because I do a lot of work in the aura. However, it also means if I am ever working along the side, I have to bend over slightly.

With the Chrysoprase, a great deal of work was done throughout her body, with much circling everywhere. This told me that the body realized that it must counterbalance all the work that was done at the head with work on the body.

This is one of the beauties of working with different mini-gemandalas in the same session. Each central gem reflects back to the body's intelligence a different perspective of what is going on. This way, the higher intelligence can figure out how best to support healing in the target area or issue.

At this point, my client mentioned she was feeling freer from tension and relaxed enough to sleep. She said "it feels so good!"

Jiggling

Soon, we encountered some jiggling movements that let us know we met some disturbance in her field, but the disturbance was minor enough that we did not need the spray. Only a few circles were needed to clear it out. Had the jiggling continued or had it felt sluggish, then I would have used the Energy Clearing spray. I tend to give a disturbance a few circles first, just to see if the body can work out the trouble on its own before I bring in a spray.

Work at the Root Chakra

Then, the gemstone therapy centered over her root chakra, and at this point we saw a plunging movement. Plunging is like an energetic massage. It helps the target area release unwanted energies of various kinds such as tension, stuck emotions, outdated beliefs, and toxins.

This was followed by circling, which helps re-collect and bring forward information. And then spiraling, which helps disperse whatever is being held in the area. Spiraling engages the rest of the body to help metabolize or get rid of unwanted energies through natural eliminatory pathways. Sometimes the dispersal goes directly into the aura.

Oval-shaped Circle and more Plunging

Next, the gems did a movement that was technically circling, despite its oval shape. Here, the body was gathering information, as though it was trying to decide if there was anything else it was ready to let go of. The return of the plunging movement indicated that yes, more unwanted energy was ready to be released.

When movements are performed at various levels of the aura, it indicates that these levels have been involved in holding the unwanted energies that are now being released.

Push away at Root Chakra

The Chrysoprase/Mother of Pearl mini-gemandala performed a push away at the root chakra. So we came back in at the root chakra with the final mini-gemandala in the physical healing pack: Green Tourmaline/Mother of Pearl. The body seemed to drink in the energy of the Green Tourmaline.

Treating the Spine

The circling that then took place over my client's head was not connected with the crown chakra. If it were, it would occur more towards the front of her head. This circling was toward the back of her skull.

I could sense that a connection was being made down the back of her neck and all the way down her spine. It seemed to extend beyond her feet. During a very gentle unlocking motion, it seemed that the spine was looking for ways to release tension in order to find a better sense of alignment with itself.

- When you apply gemstone therapy in the aura, pay attention not only to the movements the gems perform, but also to the target area. Try to identify what specific anatomy the gems are working on. This attention also helps to develop a deeper relationship with your client. The better this relationship, the more his or her energy field will trust you and allow you to come in and work with the deeper aspects of the health condition.

Targeting the Mid-Back from Above the Head
I sensed a build-up of gemstone energy at the middle of my client's back, and asked her what was going on there.

She said she had a bulging disk that had been a problem for her.

I didn't know of this condition, but the gemstones' energies revealed it. At that area, the gemstone energies were having difficulty moving through her spine, and so began accumulating there. The unlocking motion helped the tissue figure out how to get communication moving up and down the spine in that area. Green Tourmaline is specific for tissue repair.

The unlocking motion became more dramatic and was accompanied by the plunging motion. This growth in intensity let us know that this target area in her back was ready to release some unwanted energies. It just needed a bit of help.

Targeting the Mid-Back from the Front
Next, the gems moved to the front of her body and did circling, holding, and plunging. As the gems moved to the front of her body, they remained connected to the target area.

It's helpful to always pay attention to the target area to help you distinguish a true push away or let go. When the gems started moving away from her head, I wondered if they were finished. They weren't, because the energetic connection with the body remained. The gems were just trying to find another way to approach the next target area.

Plunging and Jiggling
When the plunging occurred with jiggling, I gave the body some time to figure out how to let go the unwanted energies that were causing the jiggling. It didn't, so I used the Energy Clearing Spray. It is very helpful to be able to apply gemstones almost equally well with either hand, but it takes practice.

Then the gems became still. I knew we had not encountered a blockage, because I sensed an uncertainty in my client's energy field as though it didn't know how to move the gemstones. At the same time, I was wondering, "Are we finished here? What else can I do?" Then I realize I was picking up what her energy field was thinking. What do we do next?

In time, her energy field figured it out. The gems began unlocking, so we knew they weren't ready to push away. They began to work in the mental layer of her aura. Meanwhile, I continued to pay attention to what was going on in the rest of her body. I did this by listening. I also asked within myself, "Is she still in harmony? Is she still in balance?"

Then we had a genuine let go.

Client Debriefing

I asked my client an open-ended question: How are you feeling?

She said she was feeling wonderful and very relaxed.

I then asked if she noticed any difference in the tension she had been holding in her body and if she felt any physical sensations during the treatment.

She replied that she had, and named her solar plexus, back, neck, and back of her head. She was very grateful for the treatment.

The video recording stopped, but we continued to debrief the session by discussing the gemstones used and the areas of her body that we worked on.

Integration Technique

I ended with an integration technique. I also used the Spinal Health Alignment Spray along her spine since the gems had focused so much on her back. I suggested she go home with the Spinal Health GEMFormula and also Energy Clearing, because so much of the work we did involved releasing unwanted energies from target areas.

Gratitude

I thanked her for the honor of being able to assist her on her journey to greater health. Inwardly in my thoughts, I thanked the masters, guides, and teachers whom we had invited to be present for and to assist in the session.

Gemstone Care

After my client left, I thoroughly cleansed the gemstones that we used, and put them away.

Notes:

Appendix

Movements to Avoid

Proficient gemstone therapy involves the careful application of your therapy rod. You want to keep the rod pointing to the body, no matter what movement you are doing.

If your therapy rod wants to tip sideways, it may be because your client's energy field is unfamiliar with the application of gemstone therapy, or that you've uncovered a significant energetic anomaly in your client's energy field. Don't let this anomaly take over the session and start initiating erratic movements. Your first duty is to respect your client's higher intelligence and support your client's overall well-being. So, keep the therapy rod pointing to the body and moving steadily and rhythmically in the ways described in this manual.

Other types of energetic disturbances may cause the therapy rod to wobble. Wobbling is a caricature of jiggling. If this occurs, hold firmly to the rod. Allow it to jiggle, but keep it pointing to the body and under control. If you let the rod follow the wobble, you may be reinforcing the disturbance that is causing it.

Finally, do not lose control of the therapy rod. Do not let it begin moving so fast that you break the connection with your client's energy field. Do not let the shape of the movements become poorly defined, nor let your performance of these movements become sloppy. This will reduce the effectiveness of the gemstone therapy.

Practice making the movements distinct and the transitions between one movement and the next as graceful as possible, and you'll be well on your way to gemstone therapy proficiency!

Notes:

Glossary

Aura: The energy field that surrounds the physical body. It consists of these layers: the supraphysical, emotional, causal, mental, and intuitive.

Causal aura: The third layer of the aura. The energy field of the causal body, where the memory, karmic records, and information about the past, present, and future are stored.

Client: The person to whom a gemstone therapy practitioner provides a gemstone therapy session.

Cushion: A barrier of energy that the body produces when it tries to protect itself from unwanted gemstone therapy tools presented to it. The higher intelligence can also produce a cushion when it wants to guide the therapy tools to work in a particular layer of the aura.

Emotional aura: The second layer of the aura, which lies beyond the supraphysical layer. The energy field of the emotional body, where emotions are born, recorded, and stored. Also called the astral body.

Energy field: The name given to the aura as a whole, without specifying any particular layer of it. Sometimes synonymous with *higher intelligence*.

Entry window: The opening in the energy field over a specific target area that appears when your client's body is ready to receive the gemstones being presented to that area.

Gemstone therapy: The art and science of applying therapeutic-quality gems in concert with your client's higher intelligence and natural energy flows to bring greater harmony, balance, and vitality to your client's body and being. When self-applied, gemstone therapy provides a way to take responsibility for your health, by allowing you to improve the vitality of your energy field so that you can feel better and enjoy your life more.

Gemstone therapy practitioner: A person who has successfully passed the certification requirements as outlined by the Isabelle Morton Gemstone Therapy Institute.

Higher intelligence (also highest intelligence): A non-local aspect of yourself that knows more about you and your needs than you ever imagined. An intelligence center exists in every cell, organ, and system, and also at the root of every chakra. Your higher intelligence governs and oversees all of them.

Intuitive aura: The fifth layer of the aura. The energy field of the intuitive or subconscious body, which relays the perceptions, wisdom, and guidance of the higher intelligence.

Mental aura: The fourth layer of the aura. The energy field of the mental body, where thoughts are experienced and also where they originate.

Mini-gemandala: A simple circular configuration of therapeutic gemstones that consists of one central gemstone surrounded by 4 Mother of Pearl. In some cases 5 or 6 Mother of Pearl may be used. Mini-gemandalas are mounted in beeswax on a therapy rod and applied in the aura.

Organs: In gemstone therapy, "organs" refer not only to visceral organs, but also to collections of tissue with specific form and function, such as hands, wrists, knees, shoulders, hips, plus any other individual muscles, joints, endocrine glands, sensory organs, or other body parts.

Patient: The person to whom a licensed health-care professional provides care.

Personal vortex: The movement of a healthy aura around the body, somewhat like the jet stream moves around the Earth. Goes either clockwise or counterclockwise around the length of the body.

Pointing to the bone: A gemstone therapy expression. It means to point a therapy rod or therapy wand to the inside of whatever anatomy you are working on, so that the rod is perpendicular to the surface of that anatomy. It also implies that the gems are deeply connected with the area they are addressing.

Self therapy: Gemstone therapy applied to oneself.

Session: The period of time in which a gemstone therapy is given, usually about one hour. Self-therapy sessions may last about only 10 to 15 minutes or more.

Shift: An energy shift marks a significant and positive change in the way energies are flowing. Shifts can be local or affect one's views of life and self.

Still point: A deeper, more reflective state than the holding movement. During a still point, information is evaluated, examined, processed, and integrated; and therapeutic changes are made. Once a still point releases, a significant shift usually occurs.

Subtle bodies: We have 4 primary subtle bodies. They are the emotional, causal, mental, and intuitive. They surround, and protect our spiritual Self from the relatively harsh vibrations of matter, energy, space, and time. The energy fields that surround the subtle bodies have unique vibrations and manifest as layers of the aura.

Supraphysical aura: That layer of your aura that immediately surrounds your physical body. A healthy supraphysical aura should be about 6 to 8 inches (15cm – 20cm) thick.

Target area: Any identifiable location where gemstone therapy is being applied. It may or may not be the area intended for therapy, but it will be associated with that area in some way. Target areas can include injuries or any tissue that needs healing attention.

Target organ: The organ, tissue, or specific body part at the center of a circle, spiral, or vortex movement, or where gemstone therapy is focusing.

Target point: A single point on the body where gemstone therapy is applied, such as where spinning, unlocking, and pressing movements occur.

Therapeutic-quality gemstones: Gemstone spheres or rondels that meet very high quality standards for color, clarity, brightness, and cut. Only a fraction of gems available meet these standards. Every gemstone has unique quality parameters.

Therapy rod: A wooden stick topped with a wooden disk, to which gems are attached in order to be applied in the aura.

Therapy wand: A wooden stick topped with a wooden bead, through which a therapeutic gemstone necklace, bracelet, or therapy strand is passed. The string of gemstones is then wound around the stick and fastened in place. The wand is then ready to be applied in the aura.

Unwanted energy: Energies that the body and/or aura have collected that interfere with health in some way. Unwanted energies can range from benign accumulation, comparable to dust on furniture, to malicious thought forms, or "entity contamination." Gemstone therapy is effective for removing unwanted energy by using the Energy Clearing spray or the White Beryl/Turquoise therapy strand for more deeply rooted cases.

Notes:

Thank you for your interest in gemstone energy medicine.
If you'd like to learn more, please visit our website:
www.GEMFormulas.com.

Notes:

www.ingramcontent.com/pod-product-compliance
Lightning Source LLC
Chambersburg PA
CBHW060805270326
41927CB00002B/58